WEIGHT LOSS FOR WOMEN:

Tighten & Tone, Perk Up Your Assets, Drop a Dress Size and Look Great Naked. No Gym Needed!

Leanne Wiese

Table of Contents:

1) Introduction:

My name is Leanne Wiese and my goal is to get you feeling better about your health and more motivated to increase your fitness level. When it comes to fitness and weight loss, efficiency should be your top priority. Why would you want to spend unnecessary time bettering your health when you don't have to? If you could spend 45-minutes doing an efficient workout in the comfort of your own home, as opposed to travelling 20 minutes to a gym, working out there for 1.5 hours and then spending 20 minutes travelling back home, which option would you choose? If you choose the first option then this book is for you, if not then you're wasting your time and you should seriously reconsider.

As a personal trainer at an all women's gym I have seen some painful sights. Women who come into the gym day after day for hours on end, working out ineffectively and never getting the results they desire. While I can see the determination and passion in their eyes they're simply doing things the hard way. Many times I will approach these women and ask them if they would like me to train them and show them how to work out in a more efficient manner, but oftentimes the answer is "no I like my routine and I'm sticking to it." That's the problem with rituals and routines, if you get into bad ones they become VERY difficult to get out of. This is why it's important to read this book, to get yourself into good routines and stick with them no matter what!

Hiring a personal trainer can be expensive and I completely understand that. I'm not saying that everyone should get one. This is the primary reason that I started writing fitness books; to provide women with excellent health information without making them pay a fortune for it. Now I'm not saying having a personal trainer is not a great investment, it really is. Many people lack the self-discipline and personal motivation that it takes to create a schedule, eat healthy and workout by themselves, and that's totally fine. Personal trainers will give you the physical presence and the human motivation that can push you down the path to a better life. But like I said, if hiring a personal trainer is not currently in your budget then I think you will find some fantastic value in the pages ahead.

Being fit and healthy has always been an integral part of my life; it is something that I have personally identified with over the past ten years and it has become part of who I am. I try to be active every single day of my life and I try to ensure that my diet is as clean and healthy as possible. There was a time, however, when I was not healthy. I often think back to this time and reminisce about how awful I used to feel about myself. This was a feeling that I wouldn't wish upon anybody and I understand that **it's a feeling that many women have right now while reading these words.** If this is you, it's okay, I'm here to help you because I remember what it was like. I remember the feelings of laziness, little motivation, not wanting to get out of bed, deciding to eat a whole bag of chips just because they were there and I can gladly say that this part of my life is far behind me.

Now that my happiness has increased and I feel like a new woman I really want to spread the word about how fitness can enhance every aspect of your life. You will think more clearly, have better sex, be more confident, have a better attitude and quite frankly **you will just get more shit done on a daily basis!** What if when your alarm clock went off in the morning you had the energy to spring out of bed, because you were so tired the previous night that you fell asleep seconds after your head hit the pillow? What if when you got out of the shower and looked at your naked body in the mirror you could feel sexy and proud? What if you were forced to throw out most of your old clothes because you dropped a whole dress size and could no longer fit in them? What if you could lift your butt and perk up your breasts? What if I told you that you could do all of this with no gym, in the comfort of your own home? You can and it all starts in the following pages of this book, let your journey to happiness begin.

2) Fitness Motivation:

From time to time we all lack motivation, it's completely normal. We can't all be pumped up and determined to better our lives every moment of every day; that would just be plain exhausting! What we can do however is put ourselves in a position where maximizing our happiness becomes a greater possibility. The way to do this is by **developing a strict routine and sticking to it no matter what**. You know those days where you wake up after a solid sleep, eat a healthy breakfast, go for a quick jog, do some yoga, or whatever your physical activity of choice may be? Those days where you feel ready to conquer the world and achieve success no matter what obstacles you may face? We need to pinpoint the variables that make you feel this way, that make you feel the most productive and happy that you can possibly be. The next time you have a super productive day, where you feel energized and bulletproof, try to pause for a moment before going to sleep to ask yourself what you altered in your routine to cause that day to be such a success.

For me personally, I know that I need to do a few sun salutations (yoga poses) every morning when I first wake up. Next I need to drink a big glass of lemon water and do a workout that I wrote for myself the night before. After the workout I eat a good clean breakfast (normally some quinoa with brown sugar, cinnamon and almond milk and a smoothie). If I can do these four things every morning then I know that my chances of having a productive day go up drastically. Maybe you like to meditate, surf, swim, sing or take your canoe out for a paddle every morning. You should, as early as you can in your day, try doing whatever activities make you feel fulfilled and give you energy.

Being healthy and fit is more than a fad or a temporary diet; it's a lifestyle choice that requires lots of work and dedication. If fitness were easy, everyone would be fit. You need to take action when it comes to your health, you need to look yourself in the mirror and ask yourself:

Is this the body I want? Am I satisfied with how I feel about myself?

If your answer to either one of these questions is no, then you must decide to take massive action and make a significant change in your life.

For many of us it is going to take more than a sudden burst of willpower to make a drastic change. Many people will not take action until they've either had a light bulb moment or hit a breaking point. I define the former, a light bulb moment, as a sort of epiphany where everything begins to make sense in a matter of seconds. This might happen one night while your sitting on the coach watching television and you suddenly realize that being healthy isn't such a difficult thing to do. Maybe you decide right then and there to begin managing your time in a more health conscious way and you go for a 30 minute walk. Perhaps you keep this routine up and before you know it you're walking for an hour a day. This alteration in your physical routine might prompt a change in your diet and before you know it you're on your way to a healthier lifestyle.

The latter example, a breaking point, is less pleasant, but it seems to be a more common catalyst for dramatic change. Breaking points can occur in a number of ways; maybe you've had a major health issue like a heart attack, or maybe you're significant other left you because you're unhealthy and your life is falling apart. Whatever the cause of the breaking point may be, the only thing that matters is that you use this negative event and turn it into a positive form of energy that I like to call motivation. Allow the painful moments in your life to be harnessed and utilized in an effective way. Don't just take the punches that life throws at you, counter the punches and throw them right back! Don't let life beat you down, you must learn to conquer adversity and become the phoenix that rises from the ashes. I know that sounds very cliché, but I think it's a useful metaphor in this situation.

I think one of the main reasons people fail when trying to improve their fitness level is because they don't manage their time properly and they don't **write down their goals** (long and short term). By writing down your daily goals in some sort of notebook, you materialize these ideas into necessities. By writing things down you make them real. Have you ever had the experience of having to write down information (maybe a phone number or a date) in order to remember it at a later time, only to realize that by writing it down you now have the information perfectly memorized? This happens because by writing the information down you make it real, and you tell your mind that THIS IS IMPORTANT SO I SHOULD REMEMBER IT.

I always plan out my daily workouts by writing them down and sticking to them. If you're not doing this then you must start right away. Take an hour of your time and write out a monthly health/fitness goal, whether it is losing five pounds, walking 20-minutes a day for the entire month or cutting out pizza from your diet. Make multiple goals and be sure to be very specific when creating the goals. If your goal is too broad you will not be able to properly track your progress. The more specific your goal is the harder it will be to pretend that you've completed it. Humans are experts at rationalization and if your goals are too vague then you may trick yourself into thinking you've completed them, when in reality you may just be settling for a partially completed goal. Every morning when you wake up or before you go to sleep at night, write out your daily goals and stick to them. Every daily goal should be seen as a stepping-stone to completing your monthly goal.

I am giving you a head start when it comes to writing down daily fitness goals by providing you with a 4-week workout plan in this book. I suggest that you stick with the plan and really pay attention to how the workouts are structured, that way once you complete the program you will be able to continue writing new daily workouts for yourself. Use the daily workouts as part of your goal- the goal being to **complete every workout**. You should also make some daily fitness goals relating to your food and water intake. Try to eat clean and try to drink as much water as you can. If you drink any kind of pop then you unfortunately must stop right away. This is no time for complaining, you must make sacrifices and I'm being as to-the-point as I can be.

Do you want to know the primary reason that health and fitness is important to me? Could it be the way I can fit back into clothes that I used to wear in high school? Or is it the way my body looks in a bikini? Perhaps it's the increase in the number of men who approach me at bars. While these are fun benefits to being in shape and losing weight, they are merely byproducts of the ultimate health/fitness luxury. This luxury can be described as the way you feel deep inside. I'm not only talking about your self-confidence and your abs. I'm taking about how when you become healthier your brain chemistry, hormones and the entire inner workings of your body change completely. You feel totally invigorated and energized. You have a better outlook on life and you want to attack every single day with a passion that makes it seem like it may be your last day on earth. These are the feelings that await you, this is the way you can feel if you decide to take action and make a drastic change in your life!

3) Debunking Common Fitness Myths:

Here are some common myths that I figured I should discuss in order to crush any misconceptions that you may have.

Myth 1: Working Out is Much Too Time Consuming.

Reply: Yes working out can be very time consuming if you're doing it ineffectively, as most people are. If you go to the gym and run on the treadmill for an hour and a half and then spend twenty minutes in the sauna before taking a fifteen-minute shower, then I can see how you might think that working out is too time consuming. However, the reality is that you do not need to take hours out of your day to lose weight and be fit! In fact, I highly doubt that any workout in this book will take you longer than an hour, and the best part about these workouts is you don't need to go to a gym! Learning how to workout effectively is a very important skill to have and I hope you understand how to do it by the end of this book. It requires an understanding of how long you should be resting between exercises and sets, how much time you should be allocating to warm-ups and cool downs, and how much actual exercise time you need. We will cover all of this in detail later.

If by the end of this book you decide that you want to follow the 4-week workout plan, but you want to do it in a gym, then here are a few tips to keep you on track:

- Working out with a partner is fine, but don't turn going to the gym into a social affair. Focus on the real reason that you're there and pay attention to the designated rest portions of your workout and do not exceed them. Socializing is fine, but it should not be your priority at the gym.

- Hydrate often. If there's no water fountain in your gym then be sure to bring a large water bottle of your own.

- If the gym is busy and the equipment you need is being used, alter your workout/ exercises and try to avoid the crowds. If you're following the 4-week plan this shouldn't really be an issue since it requires almost no equipment at all.

Myth 2: Eating Healthy is Way Too Expensive.

Reply: This is one of the biggest lies I've ever heard and people say it a lot. I think most people say this because they want to justify the way they're eating, but the reality of the situation is that eating healthy is no more expensive than eating like crap. I also think that a lot of people are confused as to what eating healthy truly means. Eating healthy does not necessarily mean going to your local health food store and emptying your wallet on the extremely overpriced organic, natural and local food that you find there. While there is nothing wrong with doing this, it's certainly not in everyone's budget. If that is your idea of eating healthy, then yes, eating healthy is going to be very expensive. My idea of eating healthy is simply avoiding processed foods, trans fats, high sugars (especially high fructose corn syrup), high sodium and unnecessary calories (especially liquid calories). I am on a fairly tight budget and I am able to eat very healthy. I will provide you with some of the main foods that I eat, along with some recipes later in this book.

Myth 3: You Need To Pay For A Gym Membership To Be Fit.

Reply: You don't need to go to a gym! Gyms are a business and if you're convinced that you need to go to a gym to be healthy and fit, then you've fallen victim to a marketing ploy. Gyms can be very expensive and inconvenient. For the workouts in this book you will not need a gym, the only equipment you will need for some of the workouts are: a skipping rope, running shoes, a dumbbell/kettle bell and a pull-up bar (you can easily get one of these at a fitness store and temporarily put it on a doorframe). Most of the workouts require no equipment at all, why you ask? Because your bodyweight combined with gravity is enough to give you a vigorous workout. There are many benefits to not having to go to a gym. For one, you no longer need to spend extra time traveling to a gym. Two, you get to workout on your time and you don't have to pay attention to gym hours. Three, you can literally roll out of bed and start working out ASAP, which I believe is the most effective time to workout. This also means that if you're on a busy/tight schedule you don't have to worry at all. Five, you get to save money and learn how to be self-motivated!

Myth 4: Gyms Are Always A Complete Waste of Money.

Reply: I know it seems like I'm contradicting myself, but I'm trying to be as transparent as possible. Not everyone will be able to have an effective workout unless they go to a gym and there are a few key reasons for this:

1) For many people, going to the gym is part of a ritual. Once they make the conscious decision to drive or walk to the gym, they know that they must follow through with their plan. Without this ritual of leaving their residence and entering the gym atmosphere, they lose their desire to workout.

2) If you go to a gym and have a workout partner, this can be extremely motivating. If you know that your friend is going to be at the gym waiting for you, you feel more inclined to show up. If you're going to workout at home you need to be extremely self-motivated and self-disciplined. Sometimes the urge to stop working out and sit on the coach is just too much for people to fight. There are temptations all around us in our homes, we must learn to focus and ignore these distractions if we don't fancy going to a gym.

3) The fact that you must pay for a gym membership gives you motivation to get the most out of your purchase. When you exchange money for something it becomes more of a priority for you because you don't want to feel like you've wasted your money. I know a lot of people who have free gym memberships given to them by their place of employment and these people seem to rarely utilize this opportunity, as opposed to people I know who pay big bucks for a membership and go as often as they can.

4) Some people live in small residences with roommates or family. If you live with people it can be hard to have a good workout without making noise and annoying those around you.

It makes no difference if you decide to follow this 4-week program at a gym or in your home. The important part is that you follow the program and make the necessary changes in your life to become healthier. The goal of this book is not to convince you that gyms are evil, money sucking businesses that you should never go to. The take-home-point is that **you don't NEED a gym if you don't want one**. I'm trying to show you that working out at home is a viable option that you should highly consider.

Myth 5: "I Exercised Today, So I Don't Mind Eating This Cake."

Reply: This frustrates me more than anything. I hate when people try to justify eating horrible foods because they exercised that day and now they feel like they've earned junk food. Things don't just 'balance out' because you exercised, that's not how it works. I try to think about it the other way around; why would I want to waste my workout by filling my body up with fatty foods? Now I'm not saying you always have to follow a strict diet, in fact- you'll love this- having one cheat day a week or a few cheat meals a week is a great idea! You don't want to deprive yourself of your favorite junk foods; you just want to regulate how much of that junk food you're taking in. Let's be honest, there are a lot of foods out there that taste amazing, but they are also amazingly bad for you. You need to make sure the ratio between healthy foods and junk foods is weighted more on the side of the former. **DON'T WASTE YOUR VALUABLE WORKOUT TIME!** The few moments of pleasure you get from eating something fatty is not worth it.

4) Simple And Practical Weight Loss Tips:

A) Want to know a good way to wake your abs up in the morning? You only need your own body weight to do this. It's really quite simple,

-Pick a good song that motivates you and pumps you up!

-Try to pick a song that's between 3 and 5 minutes long

- Once you pick a good tune, find a comfortable area on the floor preferably with a rug or yoga mat.

- Play your song and then jump down onto the ground and into plank position.

- For a plank you want your stomach facing the ground. Put your elbows underneath your shoulders and lift yourself off the ground. Your weight should be on your elbows and your toes. Try to keep your back perfectly flat (don't sag your hips down to the ground or lift your bum really high into the air). Keep your abs tight and ensure that you have a comfortable base on your elbows/ forearms. If you want to make things easier you can move your feet wider apart. If you want to make things more difficult you can put your feet together. If you really want to make it more difficult you can wear a weight vest or a full backpack while doing your plank.

- Try to hold the plank for the entire duration of the song that you've selected. If you need to take a few breaks, that's totally fine, just make it through the entire song. This will be difficult for the first few mornings but in no time you will be selecting longer songs.

This is a good way to gauge the progress of your core strength/ endurance. The plank is a fantastic exercise because it forces your whole body to work together in fighting off gravity and keeping your stomach off the ground.

B) Never eat within two hours of going to sleep. If you're craving a snack after dinner make sure you don't eat within two hours of jumping into bed. If you eat close to bedtime then you give your body no opportunity to digest the food you've just consumed. You need to at least give your food a chance to digest before getting into bed and turning it directly into fat.

C) If you're constantly tempted by unhealthy foods, the best thing you can do is not buy them. Here's a list of some of the foods that I like to keep in my kitchen as much as possible.

- Radishes
- Green Peppers
- Cabbage
- Mushrooms
- Squash
- Asparagus
- Artichoke
- Fennel
- Collard Greens
- Bean Sprouts
- Kale
- Eggplant
- Bananas
- Oranges
- Avocado
- Mustard Greens
- Herbs
- Bok choy
- Endive
- Lettuce
- Alfalfa
- Turnip Greens
- Radicchio
- Broccoli
- Cauliflower
- Eggs
- Garlic
- Spinach
- Tomato
- Scallions
- Turnips
- Sauerkraut

- Green Beans
- Yellow Wax Beans
- Pumpkin
- Okra
- Shallots
- Fava Beans
- Coconut Oil
- Sesame Oil
- Coco Butter
- Sunflower Oil
- Avocado Oil
- Sweet Almond Oil
- Quinoa
- Chia Seeds
- Brown Rice

Like I said earlier, having a cheat day is perfectly acceptable, but I recommend buying your unhealthy foods on your cheat day only. You must ensure there are no cheat day leftovers or you will be tempted to eat these foods during the rest of the week.

D) Set small and realistic goals. By keeping yourself accountable by setting lots of short-term goals you allow yourself to feel accomplished and successful when you achieve them. While setting long-term goals is important, I would say that these long-term goals are pointless if you do not layout the strategic framework to achieve them. By strategic framework I mean short-term goals. I would suggest buying an agenda and creating weekly goals and jotting down your daily 'to-do-list.'

E) Knowing how to create workouts for yourself if you're going to be working out at home. Sometimes you will not be able to afford a personal trainer or perhaps you just don't have any friends who will workout with you. You are the only person on earth that you can truly control, so you need to make sure that you are being dependable and consistent so that your body does not suffer the consequences. The primary goal of this book is to guide you down a path to a healthier and fitter life. The secondary goal of this book is to make you more independent by giving you the necessary tools and knowledge so that you can create your own workout schedule and stick to it, FOR LIFE!

Once you get good at creating your own workouts, it becomes really fun because you get to engineer your own fitness level. The tricky part is judging if workouts are going to be too hard or too easy. Once you've read this book and completed all of the workouts, you should have a good idea of the kinds of workouts you excel at, and the kinds of workouts that you struggle with. I recommend keeping a training journal so that you can write how you feel after every single workout that you complete. This book focuses on functional strength, which I deem to be the most important and underestimated area of fitness. If you've got other exercises that you enjoy that I haven't mentioned in this book, you can just incorporate those into your workout schedule. Here is a step-by-step rundown of how I create my workouts.

1) I decide which areas of my body I want to target. For this example let's say I want to target my back, core and legs.
2) I determine how much time I have to workout. Ideally I like to set aside at least an hour, that way I have time to warm-up, workout and cool down/stretch afterwards. But let's say in this example I only have 35 minutes.
3) I select an even number of exercises that I want to do. In this example I will choose 6 exercises: pull-ups (for back), mountain climbers (for core), lunge walks (for legs), kettle bell swings (for back & core), reverse crunches (for core) and squats (for legs).
4) Now I must decide what type of workout I want to create. Do I want to do a short explosive/anaerobic set workout with short amounts of rest? Do I want to do a long timed set that will give me a good cardiovascular/ aerobic workout? Or do I want to do a combination of both? Since I only have 35 minutes in this example, I am going to create a short set workout with minimal rest.
5) Let's do 3 sets of each exercise. Pull ups are a more difficult exercise so we will only do 6 reps. Mountain climbers can be done relatively quickly so we will do 25 reps. For lunge walks we will do 10 reps. We will perform 15 kettle bell swings, 20 reverse crunches and 15 squats.

6) Now we should write our workout down on paper so that we can glance over at it if we ever forget what we should be doing. The workout on paper will look like this:

3 Sets of 6 exercises:

6 pull ups

25 mountain climbers

10 lunge walks

15 kettle bell swings

20 reverse crunches

15 squats

7) The workout has been neatly written down and we now need to determine what our rest will be. Since we want to make this workout short and intense, we want to minimize the rest. Let's do 15 seconds rest in between exercises and 1:30 rest between sets.
8) It's time to determine what we will do for warm up. Since we're crunched for time, let's do 50 jumping jacks, 5 burpees and 30 high knees.
9) Determine what areas of your body you want to stretch during cool down. Sometimes it's best to wait until the end of your workout so that you can target the muscles that have become sore. Stretching is very important for injury prevention and muscle mobility and it should never be neglected.
10) Get down to business and get that workout going!

This is a basic workout, but it shows you just how simple workout creation can be. Depending on what areas of your body you wanted to target, the exercises could have been drastically different. The key is choosing what you want the focus of the workout to be, creating a game plan and sticking to it.

They always say that you should never go grocery shopping on an empty stomach, because you may be tempted to buy more than you normally would. I always say that you should never create workouts when you are tired, because you are more likely to make an easy workout that you will not struggle at all to complete. Workouts are meant to be challenging, if you do not push your body it will never get stronger, it's really that simple. Challenge your body often and it will thank you forever. While it's important for you to follow the 4-week plan later in this book, it's also important that you pay attention to how each individual workout has been created. By understanding the creation of the workout you will be able to create your own unique and fun workouts once you have completed the program. You don't want to just keep completing the workouts in this book over and over again because you will get board and you body will get used to the exercises, hence it will hit a plateau and you will not notice any changes.

5) **Explanation of Key Exercises:**

Here I will be explaining all of the exercises that you will have to do in the 6-week program. I will do my best to explain them all but if any of them seem unclear there are certainly YouTube videos out there that can give you a more in-depth idea on how to do particular exercises.

Understanding Workout Terminology:

When reading a workout the first number is the number of sets and the second number is the number of repetitions per set. So if you see 4 x 20, that means four sets of twenty reps per set. During a set you perform every exercise in order with no rest between exercises unless otherwise instructed. Some workouts will be timed such as 3 x 1:00, 1:00 off, 1:30 on. For this workout you would be doing each exercise in the set for one minute, resting for one minute and then doing that same exercise for one and a half minutes.

The Kettle Bell Swing:

You can use dumbbells instead of kettle bells; it's just a little harder to hold onto them. Remember to start light, grip the kettle bell with two hands, let it swing between your legs, slightly bend your knees, then thrust your hips and straighten your legs simultaneously while keeping your back straight to swing the kettle bell up to eye level. Arms should be slightly bent, feet at shoulder width apart. The weight you use is totally dependent on the number of repetitions you will be doing. If you are a beginner I recommend starting with 20-25 lbs. Your arms should not be doing much work at all, they are simply holding and guiding the kettle bell, the power of your swing should be coming from your legs, hips, core and back.

The Burpee:

Start in the standing position, jump down until your chest is on the ground, do a pushup keeping your back flat, jump your legs up into a squatted position and spring yourself up into the air with your arms reaching to the sky. With practice this movement will become fluid, but it remains a very challenging exercise.

The Squat:

Squats should be performed with your feet at shoulder width apart. Put your arms straight out in front of you and keep your back straight as you lower your bum to your ankles, keeping your legs parallel to one-another. Keep your back straight and keep your weight on your heels. Once you get as low as you can, use your legs to push yourself back up to the standing position, all the while keeping your back straight and your core tight. Some workouts require weighted squats, I recommend holding a dumbbell in each of your hands, with your arms straight when performing weighted squats.

The Mountain Climber:

Mountain climbers are great for your core. To perform, hover above the ground keeping your body horizontal. You should be on your toes and hands with your arms straight. One at a time, bring your knees towards your chest in an alternating motion. Every time both legs go in and out, you have completed one repetition.

Squat Jumps:

Squat jumps are performed just like a regular squat, but you jump into the air about 1 foot upon extension of the legs.

The Plank:

 For a plank you want your stomach facing the ground. Put your elbows underneath your shoulders and lift yourself off the ground. Your weight should be on your elbows and your toes. Try to keep your back perfectly flat (don't sag your hips down to the ground or lift your bum really high into the air). Keep your abs tight and ensure that you have a comfortable base on your elbows/ forearms.

Leg Ins:

Leg ins are done from the plank position. Once in position, bring your right knee to your right elbow, and then back. Do the same with your left side and that equates to two reps.

Pikes:

 Pikes are also done from the plank position. Simply arch your back and stick your bum into the air, returning to the plank position to complete one repetition.

The Lunge Walk:

One leg at a time, step one foot out in front of you as far as you can, while dropping the opposite knee down to the ground (don't actually touch the knee on the ground, but get as close as you can). Get a nice smooth walking pattern going as you continue to switch legs.

Wall Sits:

Put your back flat against a wall, bend your legs at about 90 degrees and hover above the ground like you are sitting in an invisible chair. Hold the position for as long as the specified time says.

Leg Ups:

 While holding onto a pull-up bar with your arms straight, bring your knees up to your chest and flex your abs.

Plank Leg Lifts:

From the basic plank position alternately lift your legs up into the air. Lift both legs once to complete one rep

Speed Skaters:

Swing your left leg behind you (in a sort of sideways lunge) and touch your right foot with your right hand, then swing your right leg behind you and touch your left foot with your left hand to complete one rep.

High Knees:

Run on the spot with your knees coming up to your chest. Each time both legs go up and down you've done 1 rep

Kneeling Super Mans:

Start on your hands and knees. Reach your right arm out straight in front of you and extend your left leg behind you. Once extended bring your right elbow to your left knee. Do the same with your left arm and right leg to complete one rep.

Hip Raises:

Lie flat on your back with your knees bent. Thrust your hips upwards so that your butt is off the ground and then lower your bum back onto the ground. Do this in a slow and controlled motion, keeping your glutes flexed the entire time.

Single Leg Hip Raises:

This is just like regular hip raises except you are going to do one leg at a time. When you are using your right leg to push your hips into the air, your left leg should be straight and vice-versa. You will find this more challenging but it really helps target each specific side of your bum.

Jumping Jacks:

Do I need to explain this one? Hop your legs in towards each other and then hop them out until they are past shoulder width. While jumping, your straight arms should be simultaneously following the motion of your legs. Essentially when your legs come together, your arms are at your side, when you jump your legs apart your arms swing up towards the sky so that your whole body looks like a star.

Squat Walk:

From the squat position, hold your arms straight out in front of you and walk to one side. Face forward and don't cross your feet. Step out to the side with one foot and follow with your other. Each step is one repetition. Try to walk in each direction for an equal number of repetitions.

Roll Back Burpee:

Jump straight up into the air, upon landing let yourself fall back onto your bum and roll onto your upper back like you're doing a reverse crunch. Roll back up onto your feet (using your arms to push of the ground if you need to) and then jump straight back up into he air.

The Reverse Crunch:

Reverse crunches are performed by lying flat on your back with your hands on the ground beside you. Your legs should be bent with your feet on the ground and you simply bring your knees up towards your chest and then back down to perform one repetition.

The Russian Twist:

For a Russian twist, sit down, lean back and let your legs hover above the ground. Rotate your core around side to side with your hands in front of you and your chest up. Let your hands touch the ground on either side of you to complete one full rep.

Jump Rope/ Skipping:

Make sure the skipping rope is the proper length. You can check this by holding the rope out in front of you, stepping on it with one foot and ensuring that the base of the handles comes up to at least your nipples. You can skip in a stationary position, or you can move around while skipping. Once you get good you can do some double unders (rope goes under you twice per jump), fast skipping, one leg skipping, heel skipping or side-to-side skipping.

The Pull-Up

Strict pull-ups are done straight up and down with your palms facing away from you. Do not swing or kip, you want to minimize the momentum and maximize the difficulty. I want you to only do strict pull-ups from now on. Get assistance if necessary when you're starting off, either from another person or by utilizing a weighted assistance mechanism found on certain pull-up machines.

U-Sits:

Sit on your bum with your knees bent and your feet hovering about one foot off the ground. The starting position for this exercise requires your legs to be straight (feet still hovering) and your arms should be straight, but off to the side as if you were trying to stop the walls from crushing in against you. To complete one repetition you must bend your knees up into your chest and clap your hands (arms remaining straight) in front of your knees.

The Super Burpee:

I want you to think 1 sit-up, 1 pushup, 1 burpee. I have dubbed this the super burpee because it is a superb exercise. Try to make this as smooth of a movement as you can. Do one complete sit-up, roll over onto your stomach and do a push up and then jump straight up into the air, like you would at the end of a regular burpee.

6) **4-Week Workout Plan For A Better Life (NO GYM NEEDED):**

Week 1: First I would like to welcome you to the workout plan. Over these next four weeks I'm going to prove to you (if you've ever doubted it) that working out at home can be extremely effective and can save you time and money! The only equipment you will need for some of these workouts is a skipping rope, running shoes, a dumbbell/kettle bell (20- 25 pounds will probably be sufficient) and a pull-up bar (I sometimes use a bar on a swing set). For each workout I've included a warm-up and a cool down. These are optional however, I do advise doing them. If you have your own ways of warming up and cooling down, then you're more than welcome to incorporate those instead. Do not alter the main sets, stick to the program no matter what! Let's dive right into it with today's workout.

MONDAY

Warm-up: 10 minute walk

Main Set: 3 X 15-20 reps of the following exercises

plank leg lifts

kneeling superman's

hip raises

speed skates

lunge walk

pikes

*Rest 20 seconds between exercises and 2 minutes between sets

Cool Down: Skip for 2 minutes and then stretch.

TUESDAY

Warm-up: 6 minutes of skipping/jump rope, then 30 jumping jacks, 30 high knees.

Main Set: Perform 4 sets of the following

20 kettle bell/ dumbbell swings

5 pull-ups

30 reverse crunches

10 push-ups

6 burpees

*Rest 30 seconds between exercises and 3 minutes between sets.

Cool Down: 6 minute walk

WEDNESDAY

Warm-up: 20 minute jog

Main Set: 6 sets of 20 reps of the following exercises

squats

mountain climbers

leg ins

leg ups

speed skaters

hip raises

*Rest 15 seconds between exercises and 2 minutes between sets

Cool Down: 2 minute skip and then stretch.

Thursday

30-minute walk/jog

FRIDAY

Warm-up: 3 minutes of skipping, 2 minutes of fast skipping

Main Set: 3 sets of the following exercises. On set 1 perform 10 reps of each, on set 2 perform 20 reps of each and on set 3 perform 25 reps of each

Pushups

Burpees

Russian twists

Squat jumps

*No rest between exercises. Rest 1 minute after the first set and 2 minutes after the second set.

Cool down: Stretch

SATURDAY

Rest day.

SUNDAY

30-minute walk/jog

Week 2: That's one week down and I hope you're enjoying the program so far. This week is going to be a little bit more challenging so prepare your body and your mind for some great workouts.

MONDAY

Warm-up: 20 lunges, 30 high knees, 40 jumping jacks

Main Set: 6 x 4:00 jog, 1:00 sprint

You get no rest on this workout; once you finish the sprint you should jump right into your next four-minute jog. This is a fantastic speed/ endurance workout and it will get you sweating in a hurry.

Cool Down: 10 minute walk.

TUESDAY

Warm-up: 2 sets of 5 squat jumps, 6 lunges and 10 mountain climbers.

Main Set: 4 sets of:

50 kettle bell swings

30 leg ups

1:00 plank

30 mountain climbers

1:30 wall sits

40 hips raises

*Rest 2:00 between sets and 20 seconds between exercises.

Cool Down: 2 minute skip and stretch.

WEDNESDAY

Warm-up: 10 minutes of skipping

Main Set: 4 sets of:

25 squats

20 single leg hip raises

30 kneeling superman's

40 high knees

25 speed skaters

50 plank leg lifts

*Rest 2:30 between sets and don't rest between exercises

Cool Down: Stretch

THURSDAY

Rest day.

FRIDAY

Warm-up: 10 minute jog

Main Set: 2 Sets of the following:

30 jump rope

30 leg ups

20 jump rope

20 pikes

10 jump rope

10 leg ins

2:00 plank

*Rest 20 seconds between exercises and 2 minutes between sets

Cool Down: 10 minute walk

SATURDAY

Warm-up: 20-minute jog

Main Set: 2 sets of:

30 double unders (jump rope)

30 burpees

20 double unders

20 burpees

10 double unders

10 burpees

* Try not to rest at all between exercises, make your transition quick and fluid. Rest 4 minutes between sets. If you can't do double unders just do double the amount of normal skipping jumps (instead of 30 double unders you would do 60 regular skips)

Cool Down: Stretch

SUNDAY

Warm-up: 6 minutes of skipping

Main Set: 30 minute jog, every 4 minutes stop your watch and perform 15 mountain climbers, 10 lunges and 6 squat jumps. Resume jogging and start your watch again when the short workout set is done.

*No rest

Cool down: Stretch

Week 3: That was a tough week, great job! Hopefully by now you're starting to understand the benefits of working out at home. I hope that you are not having any difficulty staying committed to the program. I know sometimes working out at home can be difficult and it can very tempting to skip workouts, but don't! You're better than that and you must complete this program. The more you think about workouts the harder they become, so don't think just do!

MONDAY

Warm-up: 30 jumping jacks, 30 high knees

Main Set: 6 sets of the following:

30 hip raises

40 kneeling superman's

30 leg ups

2 minutes plank

30 leg ins

40 jumping jacks

20 plank leg lifts

45 squats

*Rest 20 seconds between exercises and 3 minutes between sets

Cool Down: Stretch

TUESDAY

Warm-up:

Main Set: 3 Sets of the following:

40 jump rope

40 squats

30 jump rope

30 kettle bell/dumbbell swings

20 jump rope

20 pikes

10 jump rope

10 pullups

2:00 plank

*Rest 30 seconds between exercises and 3 minutes between sets

Cool Down: 10-minute walk

WEDNESDAY

40-minute jog

THURSDAY

Warm-up: 10 minutes of skipping

Main Set: 1 set of:

1:00 wall sit

1:00 plank

1:00 squats

1:00 kettle bell/dumbbell swings

Rest for 2 minutes

1:30 wall sit

1:30 plank

1:30 squats

1:30 kettle bell/ dumbbell swings

Rest for 2 minutes

2:00 wall sit

2:00 plank

2:00 squats

2:00 kettle bell/dumbbell swings

*Rest as instructed.

Cool Down: Stretch

FRIDAY

Rest day

SATURDAY

30 minute jog

SUNDAY

8 X 2 minutes jog, 30 seconds sprint

*Rest 1 minute between sets but don't stop during the rest. Keep your body moving by walking so that you don't cramp up.

Week 4: This is the final week; the home stretch and I know you can do it! The best part about you completing this workout program is that you should now hopefully know how to easily create your own workout plan. Like I said earlier, it's really not hard and after you get good at it, it can be a lot of fun!

MONDAY

Warm-up: 50 jumping jacks, 3 minutes of skipping

Main Set:

2 sets of

10 minute jog

50 squats

10 minute jog

*No rest

Cool Down: Walk until cooled down

TUESDAY

Warm-up: 5 minutes of skipping

Main Set: 3 sets of:

1:00 speed skipping

1:00 kettle bell/ dumbbell swings

1:00 speed skipping

1:00 burpees

1:00 speed skipping

1:00 mountain climbers

*Rest 2 minutes between sets

Cool Down: 2:00 light skipping

WEDNESDAY

Rest day

THURSDAY

Warm-up: 100 jumping jacks

Main Set:

Go for a minimum of a 1-hour jog. If you can jog for 1.5 hours that's awesome. Try to run the entire time, only walk as needed. Pace yourself and never stop moving forward.

FRIDAY

Warm-up: 4 minutes of light skipping, 2 minutes of speed skipping

Main Set:

3 sets of:

40 squats

30 hip raises

20 squat walks

10 plank leg lifts

5 squat jumps

3 burpees

*Rest 3 minutes between sets and do not rest between exercises

Cool Down: 10 minute walk

SATURDAY
Warm-up: 30 arm circles, 30 high knees, 30 jumping jacks

Main Set:
5 x 30 reps of:
kettle bell swings
squats
reverse crunches
lunge walks
high knees
speed skaters
*Rest 30 seconds between exercises and 2:00 between sets.

Cool Down: stretch

SUNDAY
Warm-up: 10-minute jog

Main Set:
10 minutes of as many sets as you can complete of:
10 squats
6 lunge Walks

3 burpees

*No rest! Set a consistent pace and try to work hard for the entire 10-minute period. Do as many sets as you possibly can!

Cool Down: 3 minutes of light skipping

******CONGRATULATIONS******

7) Healthy Recipes:

Creamy Avocado Pasta:

Serves two

What you will need:

Noodle Bowl:
2 medium zucchini (1 per serving)
1 small cucumber (1 per serving)
½ cup chopped cherry tomatoes

Creamy Avocado Sauce:
1 avocado
½ cup coconut milk
2 cloves of fresh garlic
2 tbsp. fresh lime juice
¼ cup chopped fresh cilantro
pinch of sea salt & cracked pepper
pinch chili flakes (optional)

Spiralize your zucchini and cucumber. Dice tomatoes and add to the noodles and set aside. (You can either mix everything together in a separate bowl or transfer to individual serving dishes or you can serve and mix right in your serving dish.) You can also julienne by hand or use a julienne tool but the spiralizer is really fun and easy. I highly recommend having one if you make raw noodles often- they are super easy, delicious and versatile.
Next you will prepare the creamy avocado sauce. Slice and scoop out the flesh of one avocado into a food processor or blender. Add about ½ cup coconut milk slowly and blend until desired consistency. Add cilantro, lime juice, salt and pepper. This is a great recipe to play with and come up some different variations using herbs and spices you prefer. Also the texture of the sauce can be altered to your tastes by adding more or less coconut milk. The lime and cilantro complement each other well, but as an added bonus the lime juice also helps to keep the avocado from turning brown. Top the noodles with the sauce, and serve. Top with chili flakes, sliced green onions, fresh herbs of choice, mineral salt & cracked pepper to taste.

Blueberry Blast Smoothie:

Serves one

What you will need:

In a blender, blend the following ingredients to your desired consistency:

1 frozen banana

1 cup of frozen blueberries

1 tbsp of flaxseed

1 tbsp of natural peanut butter

1 tsp of coconut oil

1 tsp of chia seeds

1 handful of spinach

1 handful of kale

1 cup of coconut water

1 and ½ cups of unsweetened vanilla almond milk

Sprinkle cinnamon as you desire

Notes- this smoothie packs a nutritional punch and the best part about it is that it tastes amazing. Drink this first thing in the morning and you will wake up in a hurry. It's got everything you need, protein, fiber, essential oils, fantastic hydration and amazing taste. You will not be disappointed when you try it.

Mango Banana Berry Sorbet

Makes one bowl.

What you will need:
1 frozen banana
1 cup cubed frozen mango
½ cup cubed frozen pineapple
2 tbsp water
½ cup fresh berries of your choice

Blend the banana, mango and pineapple in a blender or food processor. If your blender or food processor sticks you may need to add about 2 tablespoons of water. Poor in a bowl and top with fresh berries.

Enjoy anytime!

Although breakfast is my favourite meal of the day, the good thing about this recipe is it can be enjoyed at any time, not just breakfast. This sorbet is wonderfully refreshing on a hot summer day or after a steamy yoga session!

Grilled Salmon with Spaghetti Squash and Pecan Salad

Yield: Four Servings
Active Time: 30 minutes
Cooking Time: 55 minutes
Total Time: 1 hour, 25 minutes

Ingredients
- 4 wild-caught salmon fillets (Each fillet should be about 6 ounces)
- 3 cups spaghetti squash, diced
- 1 cup celery leaves
- 1 cup yellow onion, thinly sliced
- 3 cloves garlic, divided (2 crushed separately and 1 sliced)
- ¼ cup pecan halves, toasted
- ¼ cup toasted almond halves, toasted
- 1 ½ tbsp fresh lemon juice
- ½ cup fresh parsley, coarsely chopped
- 1 tbsp garlic cloves, minced
- 2 sprigs fresh thyme, finely chopped
- 1 cup unrefined virgin olive oil (divided)
- Himalayan Pink Salt
- Ground black pepper to taste
- Unrefined extra-virgin coconut oil

Cooking Directions
1. Set oven to 375 degrees and lightly grease a large baking sheet with coconut oil and set to the side.
2. Toss together squash, 1 crushed garlic clove, 1 tablespoon of olive oil, and thyme in a large bowl. Be sure all ingredients are well coated with the olive oil.
3. Dump and spread out the squash mixture onto the prepared baking sheet. Season squash mixture with salt and pepper. Bake in preheated oven for a minimum of 40 minutes. The squash should be tender. Remove from oven and allow the squash to rest.
4. Add 2 tablespoons olive oil, celery leaves, parsley, lemon juice, salt, pepper, and remaining clove of crushed garlic to a blender or food processor. Blend until all the ingredients are well combined and finely chopped. Set pesto sauce to the side.
5. Prepare your grill to your preferred temperature.
6. Coat salmon fillets with a layer of olive oil, salt, and pepper. Slowly add seasoned salmon fillets to the prepared grill (skin side down) and grill for a minimum of 5

seconds or until the fish is easily flaked with a fork. Turn off the grill and allow the fish to rest, but keep warm.

7. Sauté sliced garlic and onion in a large pan over high heat. Season with salt and pepper and simmer until the onions begin to caramelize. Mix in squash, almonds, and pecans. Simmer for an additional 3 minutes. Remove from heat.

8. Serve each salmon fillet with a side of the squash and pecan salad topped with the pesto dressing.

Quinoa Breakfast:

Serves one

What you will need:

1 cup of quinoa

2 cups of water

1 tsp of cinnamon

¼ cup of dried cranberries

1 tsp of sliced almonds

¼ cup of almond milk

drizzle almond butter as desired

Notes- boil 1 cup of quinoa in 2 cups of water until all the water has been absorbed and the quinoa is no longer hard. Serve yourself a bowl (put the leftovers in the fridge). After you have your bowl you can then put the rest of the ingredients on to add flavor. This is a simple and hearty breakfast that is a fantastic alternative to oatmeal.

Cheese & Chicken Stuffed Zucchini

Yield: Four Servings
Active Time: 20 minutes
Cooking Time: 50 minutes
Total Time: 1 hour, 20 minutes

Ingredients
- 1 pound ground chicken
- 1 extra-large zucchini, halved horizontally
- 2 cups tomatoes, peeled and chopped
- 1 large sweet onion, chopped
- 1 cup green bell pepper, chopped
- ½ cup pine nuts
- ¾ cup roasted almonds, finely chopped
- 1 tbsp garlic, chopped
- 2 cups organic tomato sauce
- 1 ½ cup cream cheese
- 2 tbsp fresh basil, finely chopped
- 2 tbsp fresh chives, finely chopped
- 2 tbsp parsley, finely chopped
- ½ cup fresh mint leaves, finely chopped
- ¼ cup water
- Himalayan Pink salt, to taste
- Freshly ground black pepper, to taste
- Unrefined virgin olive oil

Cooking Directions
1. Set oven to 450 degrees.
2. In a small bowl, combine cream cheese and almonds. Set aside.
3. Remove seeds and some pulp from each zucchini half, leaving about a ½" of pulp in the zucchini half. Diced the removed zucchini pulp.
4. In a large skillet, heat olive oil over medium heat. When oil begins to pop, sauté garlic, bell pepper, and onion for about 5 minutes or until the vegetables become tender. Stir in ground chicken and cook for 5 to 7 minutes or until the chicken is lightly browned.
5. Mix in diced zucchini, parsley, chives, and basil. Decrease heat to medium-low, and cook for an additional 5 minutes. Drain excess grease and season chicken mixture with pepper. Remove from heat.
6. Add tomato sauce, tomatoes, pine nuts, and ¼ cup mint leaves to the chicken mixture and spoon even portions

into each zucchini half. Place each stuffed zucchini half into prepared baking dish and add water.
7. Bake for a minimum of 20 minutes. Remove from oven and sprinkle halves with remaining mint and almond mixture. Return to oven and bake for an additional 10 minutes or until the top of the halves are crusty and brown. Serve immediately.

8) Conclusion/ Final Note:

It is my sincere hope that this book has benefited you and influenced you in a positive way. If it hasn't then I hope you can someday return to these pages and derive some sort of value from them. It is my life goal to increase the happiness of others in the simplest way I know, which is increasing their fitness level and getting them more active. I hope I have shown you that working out does not have to be expensive or complex. Far too many people are tricked into thinking that they need to spend a lot of money and a ton of time being healthy and fit. People make mountains out of molehills and they give up before they even give themselves a chance to succeed. You now have the knowledge you need to achieve your goals. I have shown you that being healthy and fit can easily be done in the comfort of your own home. There is no more room for excuses! Everybody has time to spend on themselves, so make the commitment, find the time and achieve the fitness goals that you set for yourself.

9) Bonus Sample:

If you enjoyed this book then I think you will enjoy the bonus sample on the following pages. The book is called "Butt Workout" and it is designed to give you the sculpted, lifted and toned bum that you've always wanted. Try out the workout plan in the book, you won't regret it!

Butt Workout (6-Week Plan):

The Best Butt Workout Guide And Butt Workout Routines To Give You The Lifted Butt You've Always Wanted

Leanne Wiese

Copyright/ Disclaimer Information

This book is not intended as a substitute for the medical advice of physicians. The reader should regularly consult a physician in matters relating to his/her health and particularly with respect to any symptoms that may require diagnosis or medical attention.

Cover Page Image Attribution:

http://creativecommons.org/licenses/by/2.0/

Table of Contents:

Foreword By: John Mayo

When my girlfriend asked me to write a forward for her book I was a little hesitant due to the specific subject matter. The topic of health & fitness is my true passion, but this particular book seemed a little bit too feminine and specific for my liking. Leanne assured me that I would approve of the book and after reading it for myself, I must admit that I do. As a man I had never really taken women seriously when I'd hear them commenting on men's asses, I had always thought that it was only men that cared about the shape of a woman's behind, but I guess it's a two way street!

Leanne is a true fitness fanatic. She is competitive, strong, focused and determined and as her boyfriend I have no problem saying that she has a great bum. She is a master when it comes to exercising in a way that really works her lower body, causing her bum to lift and creating fantastic shape. It's really no secret that men are attracted to women with nice asses, it's just in our nature. The workouts featured in this book are sure to give you the ass that you've always wanted.

Leanne is a certified personal trainer and creating workout programs is what she does best. She personal trains out of a gym that is strictly for women and her female clients have all seen results after being trained by her for only a few months. Leanne has taught me many of the exercises in this book and she has put me through nearly every single one of the workouts. This book receives my stamp of approval and I'm not just saying that because I'm dating the author. See for yourself, try the program, challenge yourself and get the ass you've always wanted!

Introduction:

Are you ready to get the ass of your dreams? Do you want to lift your booty up in a way that seems to defy gravity? It's no secret that men find a woman's bum to be a critical feature in determining her attractiveness. I'm not trying to degrade women; I'm just stating facts. Now ladies, I'm going to be honest with you, getting a toned butt with that natural perk and lift is a difficult thing to do. It requires discipline, focus, exercise and a proper diet. I will provide you with everything you need to know in the following pages. We will discuss dieting advice, the best exercises for getting a lifted butt, an in-depth 6-week workout plan and there will be 4 fantastic fitness tips dispersed throughout the book.

This isn't going to happen overnight. Unless you are one of the lucky few of us with fantastic ass genetics, getting the ass of your dreams is going to be a lot of hard work. As a side note to all those abovementioned ladies with lucky genetics, be wary; your amazing butt is not going to last forever without proper maintenance and if you've never really had to work for a killer booty then you probably don't truly appreciate it like someone who has. This complacency can lead to the loss of your lifted butt, so be careful!

Unbeknownst to some, having a big bum is actually healthy for a woman. Carrying weight in your back as opposed to your front is much better for your posture. Also, if you have a muscular booty it can boost your metabolism, which can help you burn fat and loose weight. Gaining muscle anywhere on your body will boost your metabolism, but why not gain that muscle in an area that's both easy to target and sexy?

Health, fitness and working out are things that truly excite me and bring immense joy to my life. I love sharing my passions with others and writing is my preferred avenue for conveying my knowledge and expertise. I have a strict daily routine that I always follow and if that routine is ever broken, my body reacts negatively. The routine consists of clean eating, various forms of exercise and stretching. Many of the workouts featured in the 6-week schedule in this book are some of my personal favorites. I have also included some of my favorite healthy food recipes as well. Follow me as we take the journey to personal enhancement and getting the ass that we've always dreamed of. After reading this book you will no longer look enviously at women with lifted toned bums, rather, you will respect and understand the effort they have put into achieving it, because you will have done the same.